THE
CARE OF THE FOOT

*A Practical Text-book on Chiropody and
General Care of the Foot*

FOR PROFESSIONAL AND PRIVATE USE

BY

WILLIAM A. WOODBURY
DERMATOLOGIST

AUTHOR OF "BEAUTY CULTURE," "THE CARE OF THE HAIR AND SCALP,"
"HAIR DRESSING AND TINTING," "THE CARE OF THE HAND,"
"THE CARE OF THE FACE," "HOW TO GET THIN AND
HOW TO ACQUIRE PLUMPNESS," ETC.

Nay, her foot speaks.
        —*Shakespeare.*

G. W. DILLINGHAM COMPANY
PUBLISHERS   NEW YORK

Copyright, 1915, by
WILLIAM A. WOODBURY

The Care of the Foot

CONTENTS.

INTRODUCTORY

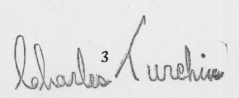

3

INTRODUCTORY.

STYLE and Comfort are not necessarily synonymous terms, but it is safe to state that a very great deal of the discomfort caused by shoes is not the fault of the style.

Many young persons and some not so young find it hard to accept a shoe quite long or wide enough. While many older persons who have realized the folly of their earlier notions, make the less painful and serious mistake of selecting shoes that are unnecessarily large.

It is the business of this little book to show in a simple, practical manner how the more common ailments of the foot may be overcome. In New York State a Regent's license is necessary to become a practicing chiropodist, so that a working knowledge of the care of the feet is no mean accomplishment for anybody.

Just what would happen if the feet were left free and unhampered we do not know. Adam and Eve are pictured with bare feet, but almost every bit of knowledge we have of man shows him with some sort of foot protection—and apparently this is the result of well defined necessity and not all style, for do we not shoe horses and other animals when pressed into regular daily service?

The shoes that are made now here in America are probably more nearly than ever before adapted to the shape of the foot and the use that is expected of both the shoe and the foot.

That people do have corns and bunions and ingrowing nails and flat feet is not direct evidence against the shoes so much as it is that the wrong shape or size was worn.

I do not believe it is necessary for comfort or safety to wear some of the homely shoes we have been told are the only thing. Nor do I believe "style" or a pretty foot require some of the shapes that are made to sell.

The whole secret seems to be in selecting a shoe and for that matter a stocking that fits—the stocking rather snugly and the shoe snug enough when first put on to be free all around when worn a while without being even a little bit loose. "Breaking in" shoes is no longer necessary, as they can now be bought the shape and size for the foot that is to wear them and worn the day they are bought.

Whether you prefer so-called French, Cuban, Military, or Flat Heels, or no heels at all, is not so important from the standpoint of beauty as it is that they be a shape and height that will enable you to get about safely, gracefully and comfortably, and that they be kept in good condition.

For summer wear the shoes and stockings selected should be a trifle wider than for cold weather, as the feet are likely to swell. If the foot is stocky, select a shoe a size or two **longer** than you really need—nobody objects to a long foot.

See that the shoes are neat and trim about the ankle. Only in extreme cases need shoes be fashioned to fit a deformity. Sufficient width of sole for displaced joints or for bunions is the obvious selection.

THE FOOT

CHAPTER I.

ANATOMY OF THE FOOT.

Expressiveness of the Foot—Racial Characteristics—Structure of the Foot.

In its natural undistorted condition, the foot is almost as beautiful and expressive a member as the hand. It can be trained to do wonderful things. A ballet dancer, such as Fannie Elsler, whose music of motion extorted the ejaculation "divine" from the Concord philosopher, Ralph Waldo Emerson, reveals the marvellous strength and pliability which the foot may acquire by assiduous cultivation. Even in its ordinary function of walking, the foot's capacity for expression strikes the eye. Virgil makes her gait the most significant sign of the goddess of beauty, Venus:

"And the true goddess is shown by her going."

Furthermore, the foot may be trained to do many things that would seem utterly outside its particular province. Men and women who have lost the use of their hands have learned to write with their toes, to sew and to embroider. To box with the feet in connection with the head and fists, is not an uncommon accomplishment among Frenchmen. It is called the savate.

RACIAL CHARACTERISTICS.—Races are markedly distinguished by differences in character of the foot. The English foot is rather fleshy, but short and not so strong as it should be. The Scotch foot, high and thick, shows power and endurance.

The French foot is recorded as long, narrow, and well proportioned.

The Russian foot is peculiar in that the skin between the toes is generally webbed to the first joint. The Tartar has toes of equal length.

The Mexican Indian foot is quite short and strong, with a noticeable distance between the great and second toes.

Savage tribes, such as the Mexican peons (now a gentle, industrious people) were a few centuries ago, usually show a decided distance between the great and second toes, undoubtedly due to the spreading of these parts in climbing trees.

The feet of Americans are well formed, but inclined to be too short for the height of the individual, especially in women.

The length of the foot of a woman five feet and six inches tall should be nine and one-third inches. Such a foot should not be thick and heavy, but slender and of delicate look, though firm of skin and with a well-defined arch at the instep that should be rather more marked than that of a man.

STRUCTURE OF THE FOOT.—The human foot may be truly said to be of a higher order than that of any of the so-called lower animals in that it is constructed not only to give ease to every poise and movement of the body, but to bear this weight gracefully and to add by its own movements, as well as its own shape, to the grace or beauty of the individual.

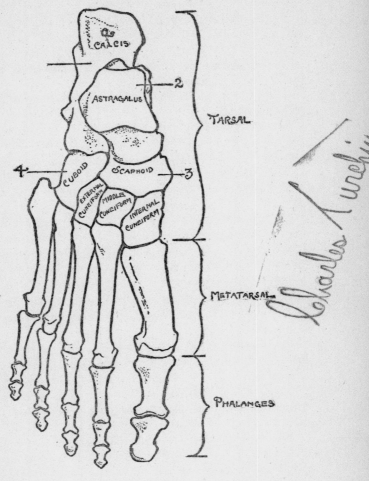

Fig. 23
THE ANATOMY OF THE FOOT

"Her feet beneath her petticoat
Like little mice played in and out"

sings the old English poet, Sir John Suckling, who understood the esthetic quality of feet as well as any physiologist appreciates their structural perfection.

Twenty-six bones, beautifully arranged, bound up together by ligaments and muscles and permitting more or less motion on one another, are found in the foot. (See Figure 23.)

The motion is chiefly on its outer or toe division and comparatively little behind the ball. Of these bones, fourteen may be said to belong to the toes, the rest composing the formation of the tarsus.

Of these fourteen toe bones, the great toe has two, the other toes three each. Back of the toes are the five metatarsal bones, numbered from the great toe one to five, making up the anterior of the arch.

The seven tarsal bones are especially named:

1. Os Calcis.
2. Astralagus.
3. Scaphoid.
4. Cuboid
5. Internal Cuneiform.
6. Middle Cuneiform.
7. External Cuneiform.

The last four of these make up the posterior of the arch. The anklebone (astralagus) is clasped on each side by the malleolus, a projection from the leg, forming what is called the ankle joint.

Architecturally studied on its inner aspect, the arch is found to rest in front on the anterior heads of the metatarsal bones; but (a point especially to remember, because of its great importance in scientific treatment of the foot) chiefly on the metatarsal of the great toe, and on the os calcis or heelbone behind. The astralagus is the keystone of the arch. (See Figure 24.)

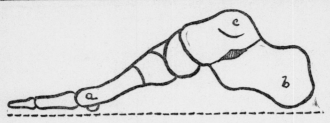

Fig. 24
THE ARCH OF THE FOOT
a=Metatarsal   b=Os Calcis   c=Astralagus

Ligaments, or strong bands, hold this marvellous piece of mechanism together and thus make it capable of upholding the weight of the body, yielding only a little as one moves, without giving way.

If we stand on one foot, the arch flattens and lengthens. If we rest the foot or dangle it over a chair, the curvature increases.

To have one leg on the floor and the other crossed over its knee gives each foot temporarily a different arch. And so in walking, as the foot is raised, by the action of the muscles, the curvature is immediately increased.

This arch is practically developed to its proper adult form about the sixth year of life; being more or less flattened during infancy and early childhood. Connecting it with the metatarsus, the great toe has but one joint, while each of the smaller toes has two.

From what has been said of the architectural relation of the great toe and the heelbone to the arch as a whole, it will be seen that in walking the chief work of the foot, running along a straight line from heel to great toe, falls upon the latter.

The great toe ought, therefore, as Professor Herman Meyer of the University of Zurich demonstrated over fifty years ago, so to lie, when on the ground, that the line of the axis, a line drawn straight through it, backward, would come out at the very centre of the heel. This is the position of a great toe on a perfectly sound foot as exemplified in the illustration Figure 25.

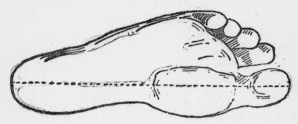

Fig. 25
THE AXIS OF THE FOOT

While insisting on the importance of the great toe, and the special care it should receive, the writer does not mean to minify the value of the smaller toes, or detract from the attention that should be paid to them likewise. They have their uses.

One of these is the giving of side support to the foot, when standing. Another is in walking, to bend in such a way as to press firmly against the ground; in this, too, giving a side support to the foot. The peculiarity about the walking curvature is, that the first joint bends upward strongly, while the second is hollow above. This would give to the smaller toes, if one went barefoot, a little grip on the ground such as is taken by the claws of a bird when walking or hopping about.

In order to ascertain the exact character of the arch effect, the chiropodist should have the patron place the bare foot firmly, but naturally, without undue pressure, on a sheet of paper that has been previously blackened with the smoke of burning gum of camphor. The imprint thus made will give a fairly indicative outline as to the perfection of the arch or its deviation from perfection.

A broken-down arch, if complete, gives an outline of the entire sole of the foot, showing the more or less elliptical imprint of the ball of the foot; the dividing line between the round impression of the heads of the smaller toes and the pear-shaped impression of the great toe; the rounded area of the heel, and a line at the outer border of the foot, more or less pronounced, which con-

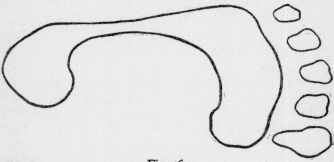

Fig. 26
THE FOOT PRINT

nects the imprints of the heel and the ball. A good idea of this impression may be obtained from Figure 26. The practitioner, when he has taken several hundred of such arch impressions, will very likely have become such an expert that he will hardly need to take them; the eye will tell him, sometimes at a glance, just what the matter is with the patron's arch, and what should be done to correct it.

In outline the foot from its inner side should appear practically as shown in Figure 27.

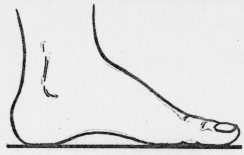

Fig. 27
THE NATURAL ARCH

If the arch has become flattened, the bones of the foot spread apart and sink down, so that the entire sole of the foot either touches or almost rests upon the floor. Such a foot is shown in Figure 28.

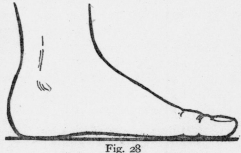

Fig. 28
THE FLATTENED ARCH

This sinking of the arch varies, of course, with each individual. If after walking for a while, one has a continual dull ache in the foot, particularly the outer side of it, and a corresponding stitch in the calf of the leg, this is a warning that the ligaments of the arch are loosening, and that the arch is likely to fall. Specific cause and treatment will be given later.

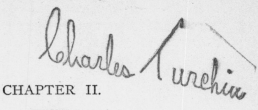

CHAPTER II.

SHOES.

Ancient Shoes: the Sandal, the Buskin—The Mocca-
sin—The Chinese Shoe—The Chiropodist as a Shoe Expert—Meyer's Reformation in Shoe Construction—Characteristics of a Proper Shoe—Children's Shoes.

FAR more than any other part of the body the foot is
affected by its covering. Every chiropodist should be
an expert on shoes, knowing the subject from beginning to end. The footgear of the ancients shows a much
clearer understanding of the rights of the foot as a member of the body than we somewhat self-appreciative
moderns appear to possess from the kind of foot cov-
erings we generally wear—to our constant discomfort
and often to the serious impairment of our health.

It might almost be said that one good reason why
Egypt flourished, and Rome stood so long, was because
their inhabitants kept their feet so well; so uncramped;
so able to support the rest of the frame in comfort, with
ease and with power.

Study the illustration (Figure 29) of an Egyptian
woman's foot, and note how the simple, light sandal affords ample protection to it against injury below and
yet allows it free play above. Would anything in foot-
wear have been more fit in a climate mostly warm and
dry, like that of Egypt?

Mark the finely arched instep and the straightness of
the toes. Such feet were almost as beautiful as hands,

and merited all the care they received. They never had corns, and only by accident callosities.

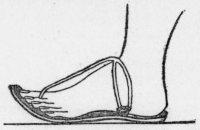

Fig. 29
THE ANCIENT SANDAL

Illustration 30 gives a fairly good representation of the old Roman foot covering called the *cothurnus,* or buskin. This was laced not overtightly (for that might interfere with circulation) over only the *root* of the *toes,* permitting even more free play than did the sandals of those pedal digits.

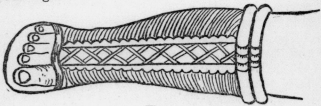

Fig. 30
THE ROMAN BUSKIN

The Roman buskin had a sandal sole made to fit the foot, instead of the foot being forced to fit the sole. Compare, too, the evenness in length of those noble Roman toes, and their *straightness,* with the irregularity of the modern foot with its one bulgy lop-sided big toe and four curlycue runts beside it.

On the ordinary Roman sandals, the thongs or strips of a thinner, more pliant leather, separated the toes and strapped the sandal to the foot, to keep the toes from leaning on or overlapping each other. Feet, thus dressed, gave off their perspiration naturally, and did not hive it up to become offensive in odor and productive of softness of the skin and of ultimate disease.

It is pleasant to note that we are beginning now, in the raising of our children, to realize the value of sandals; and it is to be hoped that this fashion, which allows the feet to grow naturally and spread properly, will continue to spread until it reaches to adults.

For men and women who spend the summer in country places or at the seaside the wearing of sandals in summer and as late into the fall as comfortable would be extremely beneficial. All athletes, whether practicing in the gymnasium or engaged in exhibitions or playing any game, except football, would be immeasurably benefited by a return of the sandal of the ancients. To golfers particularly, with the undulant character of most golf-links, the sandal would be a boon.

The American Indian covered his feet entirely with soft leathern mittens called moccasins. It would be well if these replaced the modern "sneakers" whose soles, being made of rubber impervious to perspiration, render them pernicious to the health of the feet. Pliable leather is the best protective foot covering in a cold climate. The Esquimos make their boots of skins, lining them with fur and eiderdown, and for these Arctic explorers invariably cast aside the stiff boots of civilization.

Wood, instead of hard leather, is used to protect the soles in many countries.

From time immemorial the Chinese have worn shoes having wooden soles lined with soft material and cloth

uppers in slipper fashion, which give the feet considerable freedom of movement, and consequent immunity
from corns.　(See Fig. 31.)

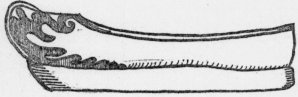

Fig. 31
THE CHINESE SHOE

But even in wise old China, Fashion, that teeming
mother of many deformities as well as absurdities, has
decreed that certain feet should be compressed to as
great an extent as possible, limiting, however, this
cruel and hideous folly to the girls of the aristocracy,
who were regarded as toys, rather than creatures with
souls demanding activity in service, and whose helplessness, therefore, was an ostentatious proof of the hus-
band's ability to afford such a luxury.

The method of doing this, which is undertaken almost
from birth, entails constant pain throughout girlhood.
By the tight bandaging, the bones are displaced upward
so as to render it short along the line of the sole and
apparently small, though the actual size of the foot, thus
distorted, remains about the same.

Carried to extreme extent, this practice renders the
Chinese belle a cripple, able only to hobble ungrace-
fully, and sometimes, when fatness arrives, necessitating
her being lifted around by servants, a pitiable piece of
feminine furniture, to whose helplessness the European
or American woman but feebly approaches with her
"French heels" and "hobble skirt."

There is no evidence in their literature that the ancients experienced such afflictions as bunions or corns.

It was with the advent of the modern shoe that all forms of foot distortion and foot-disease appeared, and with its spread that these multiplied until a perfectly shaped and perfectly healthy foot is a greater rarity than anything to be found in an anatomical museum.

Even shoes of our grandfathers' days, being custom made, were not so likely to cause abnormalities of the feet, but the recent shoes, manufactured in fixed styles and built on lasts peculiar to each manufacturer, have cut a terribly wide swath of havoc, making the chiropodist or foot-doctor an increasing necessity in our scheme of civilization.

When this highly important specialist first made his appearance, not so very many years ago, he was looked at askance as a cheap faker who gave only temporary relief. Unfortunately, this was not only true in most cases, but still worse, his treatment often caused irreparable damage.

And to-day, there are still many deplorably ignorant persons presumptuously calling themselves pedicures, and practising chiropody under license from the various States. As Dr. Kahler, who had the honor of attending to the sore feet of Abraham Lincoln, with just indignation remarks, these quacks, "ignorant of anatomy and incapable of performing a delicate operation, possessing only a few salves and the knowledge of some powerful acids or astringents, and often doing more harm than good, have brought the profession of chiropody into contempt, and to them are applied such names as corn-doctor, etc."

Accordingly, every earnest and honest would-be chiropodist should first understand the Anatomy of the Foot,

and, second, should study the make of shoes and be able
to instruct patrons just what kind of shoe to wear; other-
wise, only temporary relief, not cure, is the result, and
the foot-doctor, instead of being a desirable citizen and
an honor to any community, is a cheap charlatan whose
practice is to keep persons continually coming to himself
or to somebody else, as patients, instead of curing them
and thus converting them into active advertisers of his
probity and skill.

There are, however, reliable and conscientious chirop-
odists, and when one is found it is a good plan to visit
him at least once in every six months and have the feet
examined, just as it is a good plan to have one's teeth
examined that often by a reliable dentist.

If one has very fine or tender feet a visit every three
months, instead of semi-annually, would be advisable.
Even for persons possessing comparatively healthy feet,
to have them pedicured as often as they have their hands
manicured would be well worth the expenditure of time
and money.

THE RIGHT KIND OF SHOE.—It stands to reason that
no two pairs of feet are exactly alike. Therefore, the
shoes of modernity, manufactured by wholesale according to set forms, would inevitably cause mischief to
some feet, even if the said shoes were built along the
general natural lines dictated by the foot's architecture.

So, inasmuch as comparatively few can afford to have
shoes made especially to fit their feet perfectly, there is
all the more reason why shoe-manufacturers should
endeavor to seek such guidance from a study of anatomy as would enable them to build shoes which would
average a fair conformity with nature's clear intention,
and so create the least amount of mischief possible.

But, as pointed out more than fifty years ago by Dr. Hermann Meyer, the pioneer in the arduous field of reforming shoe-manufacturing methods, this is not done, as it ought to be, either universally or even locally to any extensive degree. Ignorance, intensified by fashion, has dominated, and in consequence the feet, the foundation of our physical superstructure, have suffered and will continue to suffer.

In the illustration (Fig. 32) of a perfectly normal child's foot, it will be noticed that a straight line drawn through the middle of the big toe emerges at the centre of the heel, and the same will be noticed in the illustration (Fig. 25), which is that of a healthy natural adult masculine foot. But in the feet of most adults, owing to the shoes they have been wearing, there is a marked deviation, the great toe having either sprawled outward or crawled inward onto other toes.

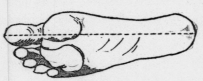

Fig. 32

NORMAL FOOT OF A CHILD

The chiropodist, therefore, after making a drawing of the patron's naked foot on paper, running the pencil lightly into the indentations indicated by the toes, should find whether the medial line of the great toe corresponds with that of the outer surface of the heel. (See Fig. 33.)

There is then before him the problem of coaxing the great toe into line again, if it has taken an abnormal position or has abnormally grown outward.

Where the curvature is inward, plugs of cork, prefer-ably wrapped round with soft cloth, are to be inserted;

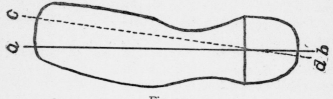

Fig. 33

THE MEDIAL LINE

ab=improper medial line   cd=proper medial line

the size of the plug should be increased gradually, say, week by week, and the kind of shoe to be worn must be not only roomy at the toes, but should be considerably longer than the toes.

If, on the other hand, the toe has sprawled outward, a soft cotton bandage, holding it pretty tightly, should be worn and the shoe should be narrower across the toes (see Fig. 34), but, as before, a little longer, so that the toe may have opportunity to straighten forward. The

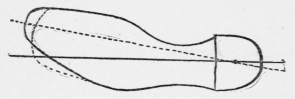

Fig. 34

SHOE TO CORRECT SPRAWLING GREAT TOE

stocking in this latter case should clasp the forepart of the foot somewhat more snugly than usual.

This slight elongation of the shoe beyond the toes not only affords fair play to them, and helps their general health, but it adds grace to the looks of the feet, especially if they be naturally broad. A short, thick foot, as has been said before, can be made to look more graceful by the selection of a shoe somewhat longer than is needed for an exact fit.

Dr. Meyer did not succeed in getting the manufacturers of his time in Europe to adopt his ideas to any noticeable extent, but his treatise, translated by John Stirling Craig and published by R. T. Trall & Co. in 1863, stimulated study of the foot in this country and led some makers of shoes to try his methods. They appear to have been discouraged, because not enough persons among the general public had sufficient understanding to appreciate the reform and by their patronage make it pay.

Some of Meyer's ideas, however, had taken partial hold of the public, particularly his approval of the so-called congress shoe, in the matter of substituting elastic at the sides for lacing. But the popularity this kind

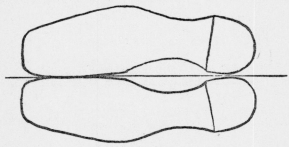

Fig. 35
SHOES IN THE MEYER STYLE

of shoe once had was very likely due to the ease with which it could be put on and drawn off, rather than to the higher hygienic quality.

Recently, however, there has been considerable attempt to restore the general shape of shoes approved by Dr. Meyer, a shoe that is comfortably broad and that appears to turn inward (see Fig. 35), but the value of this has been nullified in great measure by making it too narrow at the side next the smaller toes. We are speaking now of men's shoes. Reform in the footgear of women is a more stupendous task.

Objection may be offered that the wearing of these shoes of uncurved shape might eventually lead men to turn in more in walking or become "pigeon toed" as it is called, in their locomotion. This, of course, could be guarded against by the wearer making during the first three weeks of wear a conscious effort to toe out a little more than he usually would.

On the other hand, a slight broadening of the leather under the arch of the foot would take away the look of extraordinary incurvation and would perhaps add not a little to ease and grace in movement, and a slight extension of the toe part, as indicated in Fig. 34, would also add to its appearance. Where the instep is at once high and thick, such broadening would, of course, naturally suggest itself as fundamentally proper in the making of a shoe.

In advising a patron as to the kind of shoe to buy, the things to dwell upon with polite insistence are:

1. Sufficient width of sole.
2. Sufficient room for toes.
3. Sufficient lowness of heel.
4. Sufficient elasticity over instep.

And in case of soreness or crookedness of toes, as intimated previously, extra length in the toe part should be advised, until the condition has been permanently rectified. This does not exceed in any direction; it does not mean a shoe in which the foot slips about as in a slipper, except that in the point of length the shoe may extend considerably, which, while doing good to the toes, also adds to the shapeliness of a shoe's appearance.

The shoe should fit rather snugly to the foot. The foot should not be cramped, but firmly grasped by its leathern envelope. If the shoe is too large, the foot slides to and fro in it, which not only causes discomfort and tired feet, but induces corns and callosities, and even inflammations that require weeks to overcome.

It is equally true that a tight shoe, so generally worn, especially by women, is quite as harmful, if not more so, as a shoe that is too large for the foot. Tight shoes cause not only foot-ache, but lead to all kinds of troubles, such as corns and bunions, and also induce diseases of the blood vessels of the lower limbs, pain in the calves of the legs, headache and, in some extreme cases, trouble of the eyes.

Normal shoes, as before stated, should fit snugly, but should allow plenty of room for the toes. They should also give support to the arch of the foot by having a heel of medium height. High heels are injurious to the health of any wearer and a torture to many.

The weight of the body should be so distributed to the ball and heel of the foot that standing should be comfortable and walking a matter of easy grace, even under unusual strain, if such be not repeated too frequently.

The toe of the shoe should never be anything but of the shape of that part of the foot, slightly narrower than the bare or stockinged foot in standing. The shape of the shoe should conform to this and not be boxed or raised so that the cramped toes overlie one another.

A common-sense shoe can be made as beautiful as any

other, and its comfort will conduce to health and prosperity, for it may be truly said that one who has chronic trouble with his feet is heavily handicapped in the race of life.

A short, thick foot can be made to look more graceful by the selection of a shoe somewhat *longer* than is needed for an exact fit.

Remember that only in extreme cases of deformity shoes need be fashioned to fit that deformity. In average cases the foot after treatment should be confined in a shoe made according to the natural method, but a shade larger than if the deformity were not present.

For displaced joints and bunions a shoe considerably larger than the foot should for obvious reasons be worn at first; but, as the displacement disappears or the bunions give signs of cure, the size of the shoe should be correspondingly lessened. There are cases where, on the road to recovery, the patron may properly be advised to change the shoes several times in this way.

The ideals to be sought in a shoe are three:

1. Comfort.
2. Beauty.
3. Durability.

Here every chiropodist is going to meet his chief obstacle, particularly in dealing with feminine patrons, and frequently with men.

Style, a word derived from the sharp-pointed instruments used by the Greeks and Romans as a pen, and from which the Italian word, stiletto, the weapon of assassins, is in turn derived, has indeed been for years a weapon wounding thousands and thousands of people.

All women really wish for beauty, but the obsession of the majority seems to be that one cannot have beauty unless one is in style.

The truth is that any style, however fascinating, which in any way deforms the natural shape of any member of the body and thereby interferes with free play of functions, is contrary to the Law of Beauty, and should be religiously shunned by women for their own sake, and the sake of their children, or the children they may have if their womanhood arrives at full bloom and fruitage.

The wisest book in the world declares that the body is the temple of the living God. Now, the foundations of that temple are the feet. If these foundations are impaired, the whole temple may totter, and the light within the dome, the mind, be extinguished.

It was proved by the world-famed surgeon, Brown-Sequard, that the weight of the body, improperly thrown on one man's great toe, unbalanced his mind to a violent degree. To effect a cure a bisecting of the nerve was necessary.

The mysterious connection between the nerves of the feet, practically those of the great toe, and the brain, is now known, though not yet fully understood. But it might be hinted that one cause of many persons going astray mentally—and morally—lies in the ill-treatment of the feet from childhood up.

Mothers ought not to let their children begin to walk as early as they do; ought never to cramp the growing feet or stuff them into "stylish" shoes; *ought to take their children early to a first-rate chiropodist and faithfully follow his advice.*

In childhood the bones of the foot are soft and pliable. Machine-made shoes, bought for sake of economy, are an outrage on the helpless little one, and also entail extra expense in many ways as life goes on.

Every child is entitled to have a shoe in which the

foot can grow naturally. Anything else is an abomination.

If this reform can be started and maintained, in one generation crooked toes, corns, inverted nails, swollen joints, and bunions will virtually have disappeared.

If your patron is a wife and a mother, talk to her earnestly about baby's feet. Every mother whose feet have been a torture to her in any way will appreciate this, and, even though she may wilfully continue to suffer herself, and for the sake of wearing "stylish" shoes refuse to be cured permanently by you, she will nevertheless in ninety-nine cases out of a hundred have loving sense enough to desire that her children be set right as to their feet and started well, to that extent, in the race of life.

CHAPTER III.

THE CARE OF THE FEET.

Change of Shoes and Stockings—Bathing—Nail-Trimming—Advice for Patrons.

SHOES should be changed every day to save both feet and shoes, two pairs of shoes as near alike as possible being ordinarily sufficient. This alternation helps each pair to hold its shape, as well as to last much longer.

Alternation of socks or stockings from day to day, like alternation of shoes, is a good plan. The stockings, when removed, should be turned inside out and hung up to get well aired. They may be worn three times without washing. If they are not thus changed, clean ones should be put on at least three times a week. If it is convenient, or one's purse permits, a change at the end of the day for evening wear is advisable.

Frequently it rests the feet to rub them with a soft towel, or special footcloth, expose them to the air for a few minutes, and then don the evening socks. In all this we are speaking of comparatively normal feet.

When one has particularly sweaty feet, special remedies for which condition will be given later, a much more frequent change of stockings naturally suggests itself. But one should not, without the sanction of his chiropodist, switch from one kind or one thickness of the same kind to another.

STOCKINGS.—Stockings of which the toe section is white or cream white are preferable. The tops may be

29

of any fast color the fancy chooses. The dyes of colored stockings irritate the skin and often cause ulcers or soft corns by setting up inflammation between the toes.

Stockings should not be loose. When they grow so by frequent use and washings, they should be discarded. Loose stockings on tender feet by bunching in places cause irritation, and may produce inflammation if persisted in. Even if the creases do not seem at first to threaten any evil results, they cultivate the ground for corns and callosities. Stockings ought to fit snugly like a glove, but to possess elasticity enough not to interfere with the foot's expansion in motion.

Stockings are sometimes made with a special compartment for the "big toe"—the toe of honor, on which the burden of walking is thrown. In some cases, the use of such is to be particularly advised, and, if it could be made practicable, doubtless the whole stocking might be well converted into a foot-glove, with separate places for each pedal digit.

Heavily darned socks are just as deleterious as those with holes at the toes. Both kinds discomfort and irritate the wearer unless the feet are unusually tough.

It is desirable to have rights and lefts in stockings, though it is hard to persuade patrons to do so.

If the feet are tired and swell at night from too much standing, they should be bathed in hot water to which several tablespoonfuls of sea salt or even common salt have been added, and then be well dried and bound with white flannel bandages.

If the feet are cold, the bath should be followed with bandages of red flannel, or they should be rubbed with cologne spirits, witch hazel, or rum.

Upon arriving at home after the day's toil, it is well to rest the feet by putting on slippers with lower heels than in the shoes worn during the day. "Slippered ease" is as hygienic as it is sybaritic.

For persons who have· sedentary occupation, a foot-rest, or cushion several inches above the floor, is advisable. This is particularly so when the floor is of stone, or cement or tiling, as in many business places, or when it is of wood, but has been exposed to cold or damp air. Many carpets retain dampness. Any floor covering that cannot be often taken up and thoroughly cleaned is dangerous to health.

A fine foot bath for tired feet is made by adding the following to the simple hot foot bath:

FOOT BATH

℞ *Alum* .... ½ *oz.*
   Borax .... *1* "
   Sea Salt .... *1* "

Tender feet may be rubbed to advantage with witch-hazel, to which spirits of camphor have been added, one or two teaspoonfuls to four ounces of the former. Also to rub a little pure olive oil into tender feet, as well as upon dry and cold feet, at night after the bath is beneficial.

NAIL TRIMMING.—The nails of the toes should be trimmed at least once every two weeks. All calloused skins should be very gently scraped off or ground down with a pumice stone after the bath.

The nails should be cleaned of dirt and accumulations, taking care not to injure the cuticle under the nail, since such injury will cause them to ingrow just as cutting them too short will.

The nails should be cut squarely and not rounded as are the finger nails. The nail of the large toe should be cut concave, that is, closer to the toe in the centre than at the sides.

Dead cuticle or scales of scarfskin or epidermis should be scraped away with a blunt orangewood stick or cuticle knife, taking care not to injure the skin or make it bleed, since this invites poisoning either from stocking dye, if one is foolishly wearing dyed socks, or from the dirt which accumulates in the shoes combining with decomposing sweat.

All wounds made in pedicuring should be cleansed with an antiseptic solution at once and be covered with antiseptic absorbent cotton.

ANTISEPTIC SOLUTION

℞   Carbolic Acid (pure) .... 1 dr.
    Glycerine .... 4 dr.

Mix and apply with cotton to wound. The above solution may be used on such wounds, or a solution of boric acid, 10 grains to each ounce of water, may be substituted.

Specific treatment of diseases of the foot will be described later.

If the feet are naturally weak and cold more or less of the time, much can be done to bring them into a healthy state by bathing them every night in a hot water and sea-salt mixture made as already described. While the feet are in the bath, they should be scrubbed vigorously with a fairly stiff nail- or hand-brush to arouse the circulation, and by the pressure of this increase of blood to the parts to invite better nourishment to the skin, which before long will become thicker and more able to resist sudden changes of temperature.

Cold feet are often the result of overactive brain work. If this is the cause, the life of the patron should be regulated, and outdoor exercise and calisthenics insisted upon. If the cause of this uncomfortable condition is due to any other physical disturbance, the patient should be sent at once to a physician for proper medicinal care.

Advice for Patrons.—You may truthfully tell your patrons in an incidental way the following facts:

Sore feet hasten the advent of old age.

Diseased feet cause premature grayness.

Every long-neglected corn may be the seed of a dozen gray hairs.

Shoes too small, or improperly made, cause injury to the feet, sometimes permanent.

The story of injured feet writes itself in wrinkles on the face.

High heels cause weak knees.

Weak knees pave the way to nervous breakdown.

Wearing of improper shoes indisposes one to take proper exercise.

Lack of proper exercise invites either adiposity or consumption.

Pressure of pain in any part of the body, long continued, seriously mars the expression of the face, disturbs and sometimes ruins the disposition, and may upset the brain at last.

CHAPTER IV.

CHIROPODY.

The Necessary Instruments—Preparation of the Feet
—Treatment of Hard Corns: By Knife Alone; Medici-
nal Method—Inflamed Hard Corns—Soft Corns—Vas-
cular Corns—Removal of Callosities—Treatment of In-
growing Nails—Of Bunions—Recipes—Treatment of
Flatfoot—Artificial Arches—Treatment of Chilblains—
Recipes—Treatment of Perspiring Feet—Recipes—
Treatment of Hot Feet and Cracks Between Toes.

THE instruments necessary for the chiropodist are
not many, but these few should be of the best kind.
Cheap steel instruments soon lose their cutting edges
and have to be thrown away. The repeated buying of
such makes the ultimate expense far more than when
the best are bought in the beginning.

Following is a list of what are required:

1. Nail Clipper.   4. Scalpel.
2. Nail Scissors.   5. Pair Tweezers.
3. Corn Knife.   6. Hone.
                7. Pumice Stone.

NAIL CLIPPER.—The nail clippers should be of the
best steel, with the nail-cutting or clipper curved so that
when clipping off the nail it will give the required shape.
It is illustrated in Fig. 36.

The blades should meet evenly and be sharp so that,
by bringing the handles together, the nail will be evenly
and quickly clipped off.

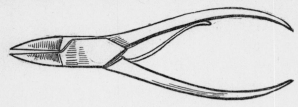

Fig. 36
NAIL CLIPPER

NAIL SCISSORS.—The scissors should be curved on the flat. The blades should be stout and short. This instrument is used to cut or trim the nails as well as pieces of loosened skin of soft or hard corns; therefore it should be of the best quality of steel. The proper kind is shown in Fig. 37.

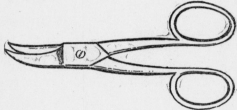

Fig. 37
NAIL SCISSORS

For hygienic reasons the so-called French lock is to be preferred, since this allows them to be taken apart and thoroughly cleansed and dried. The ordinary screw lock is hard to clean and invites sepsis.

CORN KNIFE.—This instrument is a type of razor, a short, slightly hollowed blade with one cutting edge, blunt at the end and back, where it is thickened.

The handle should be of steel, nickel-plated to insure

cleanliness. Bone or horn handles soon become loose and useless from the boiling which is necessary in the proper cleaning of all instruments, and antiseptic solutions attack them readily. The proper instrument is shown in Fig. 38.

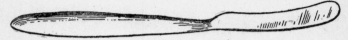

Fig. 38
CORN KNIFE

This instrument should never be used on the nails or bony callouses, for such employment soon destroys its fine, razor-like edge.

SCALPEL.—This is really a small, metal-handled operating knife which is used for paring off callous skin and soft corns, and not for cutting hard corns. It should be of the best steel, not too thick in the blade and of the size and shape shown in Fig. 39.

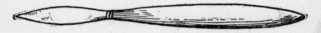

Fig. 39
OPERATING SCALPEL

TWEEZERS.—The tweezers should be of steel, with stout, well-meeting sharp points, ribbed inside of the points and outside in the handles to permit of a firm hold. They are used to raise pieces of skin or soft corns that have been loosened, or partially dissected with the scalpel, and which are to be cut away finally with the scissors. These tweezers are called Dressing Forceps, and are shown in Fig. 40.

The tweezers are also to be used to convey dressings

of small size to the parts operated on, or to crowd cotton under ingrown nails, as later described.

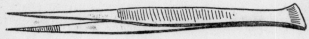

Fig. 40

DRESSING FORCEPS

HONE.—The hone to be selected for the sharpening of knives should be of the best quality. The usual barber's hone is a little too fine. An oil stone of high quality answers best. It should be about four inches long, and one and one-half inches wide. Plenty of oil should be used in sharpening, and the knife should be drawn evenly toward the centre of the hone, edge inward, first the one side and then the other of the knife. A number of strokes are needed to get a good edge. Drawing the knife away from the centre of the hone with the knife edge outward tends to give a sawlike edge.

PUMICE STONE.—At the present day pumice stone may be had in various-sized pieces of regular shape, either oblong, oval or round. It is best to purchase one of these, instead of using the rough and irregular stone, as it makes a better impression, while it does the work more effectively.

PREPARATION OF THE FEET.—To prepare the feet properly for pedicuring, they should be soaked for a few minutes in as hot water as can comfortably be borne. A little borax, about a teaspoonful, may be added to the water. It renders the latter slightly antiseptic, and helps to soften the cuticle and corns as well as the toe-nails.

Remove the feet from the bath and dry with a clean towel, rubbing *downward* toward the toes. Dry well and pay particular attention to the skin between the toes.

Moisture does not permit of good work. When the skin is wet the fingers are liable to slip nor can the instruments render as good service.

DISEASES OF THE FEET.—There are a number of diseases of the feet which the chiropodist will be called upon to treat and overcome; and to give the proper knowledge and the practical method of treatment each will be fully considered under its own heading.

CORNS.—The most common disease of the foot is the so-called corn. There are three types generally considered:

1. Hard Corns.
2. Soft Corns.
3. Vascular Corns.

HARD CORNS.—These painful, localized callosities are usually found upon the toes, particularly on the second joint of the small toe, but they may occur on all toes, and at one or both joints of each, or the skin over one or two of such joints of all the toes may alone be affected.

A corn is composed of callous skin, having a central plug of horny skin pointing downward into the sensitive layer of the true skin. The outer cuticle, or horny layer of the skin, is thickened by reason of constant irritation, or the pressure caused by shoes which are either too tight or too loose, or which do not match the shape of the foot. In tight shoes, the cause is pressure; in loose, friction; in shoes that do not perfectly fit the shape of the foot, it may be both.

As the horny layer becomes thicker, the plug beneath its central point is forced deeper into the sensitive true skin, and walking becomes a painful task, even the mere touch of the finger sometimes producing an acute ache. If the cause of the disease continues, the skin about and below the corn becomes highly inflamed, and an abscess may eventually form which at once becomes a serious condition, liable, without proper antiseptic care, to end in blood poisoning.

When, therefore, one discovers a corn on one of the toes, it should be treated at once, not simply to cut away the callous skin, but to remove the corn permanently. This will sometimes prove a tedious task, especially if the patron persists in clinging to the ascertained cause of the trouble.

It is well to tell your patron that to cut away a corn and give present relief is an easy matter, whereas to prevent its recurrence requires not only skill on your part, but the patron's co-operation. Much can be done, however, in the average case by following the methods herein given.

The foot upon which the corn has come is immersed in a hot footbath. The water should be as hot as can be well endured, since the heat by expansion of tissue softens the corns, at the same time reducing the irritation of the whole toe. The foot should remain at least ten minutes in the bath. It is then dried, and placed with the heel down upon a properly cushioned stool, which has previously been covered with a clean towel.

The afflicted toe is then taken between the thumb and forefinger of the left hand. The corn knife is held in the right, and with it the operator, gently and carefully, pares down the hard mass, working from the *centre* of the corn *outward* or *toward* himself.

Proceed in a circular manner to trim away all the callous part, until the skin becomes thin and rosy in color. Do not cut so deeply as to draw blood.

This done, apply a little carbolated vaseline to the part operated on and allow it to be absorbed.

The next step is to prevent further friction or pressure. To overcome this, cut out a disc of felt, or one or two pieces of chamois skin, about four times the size of the corn. Then cut a circular piece out of the centre of the disc of the material used, about twice the diameter of the corn.

· The disc, thus formed, is laid upon the toe with the corn at the open centre. Fasten the disc down with several fine strips of adhesive zinc oxide plaster, or paint the part over with flexible collodion, applied in several layers with a fine camel-hair brush, letting it dry and harden.

Flexible collodion can be obtained at any drug store. It forms a skin or film when painted on any surface, and is preferable to plasters, which are liable to be sweated off or rubbed off in walking.

The stocking may now be drawn over the foot and a proper shoe worn. An old shoe will be found best for the purpose, or the shoe may be cut in such a manner that the pressure over the corn is relieved. If the pad is properly put on, in nine cases out of ten cutting the shoe should not be necessary.

The pad, or disc, applied as directed, is removed the second or third day, and a new one applied. This treatment should be continued until the corn disappears, or until it fails to rebuild itself. After that the patron should look to the wearing of proper shoes.

THE MEDICINAL METHOD.—Another method of removing a corn permanently is to pare down the hard callous mass and then paint the corn with the following mixture:

℞ Salicylic Acid .... 1 gram
Tincture of Cannabis Indica......... ½ gram
Alcohol 95%........................ 1 gram
Ether 65% .... 2½ grams
Flexible Collodion .... 5 grams

A coating of this paint should be applied on the corn every day for at least a week, care being used not to paint the surrounding skin. On the eighth day, after a hot footbath, remove the collodion skin and the corn will come away with it. If it does not come away entirely, the same method is to be repeated.

Once removed, all pressure of the shoes at the afflicted part must be guarded against.

Another method is to use the following plaster:

℞ *Resin* .... 3 dr.
   Balsam of Tar........................... 2½ dr.
   Salicylic Acid .... 5 dr.

Melt the resin and balsam together over a slow fire; add the acid and stir until the mixture is even.

Then place a pad of felt, or chamois skin, with a hole in its centre over the corn. This pad should be stuck to the skin, with a mixture of equal parts of balsam of fir and resin, melted over a slow fire. Stir well, and while still warm, paint it on the under side of the felt or chamois skin, which, when cold, can be cut into discs, and a hole made in the centre.

Having fastened the disc to the corn, a little of the paste, of which the recipe has just been given, is put into the hole over the exposed corn. A quantity equal to the size of a half pea is about sufficient. This is allowed to remain in the corn for one or two nights, or until it drops off of its own accord, when the corn will come away with it. If the corn is not entirely removed, the method is repeated. All pressure of the shoe should be guarded against thereafter.

INFLAMED HARD CORNS.—If the skin about a hard corn is inflamed and tender, it is best to reduce the inflammation with hot water baths, allowing the foot to remain in the bath at least fifteen minues. Dry the skin thoroughly and relieve the corn of all shoe pressure with a chamois pad as above directed. Repeat the bath the next day and remove the corn as heretofore directed.

If the above treatment does not overcome the soreness, place a hot poultice of linseed meal about the corn overnight, removing the corn the next morning. The linseed meal is mixed with hot water till it forms a paste, then is put in cheese cloth as applied, or may be plastered over and bandaged on, the meal coming into direct contact with the corn and surrounding tissue.

SOFT CORNS.—The soft corn is, in structure, the same as the hard corn; but is found usually on the *side* of the toe where there is sufficient moisture to keep the callous skin soft.

To remove a soft corn, separate the toes with the fingers of the left hand, after the proper preparation of the foot, as described before, and remove the thick cuticle with the scissors, being careful not to make the parts bleed.

But a better or more scientific method is to employ a Toe Expander, which holds the toes apart, leaving both hands of the operator free to work with. The instrument, which is cheap, is so made that it can be held in position with a set screw; it is shown in Fig. 41.

Quite often the soft corns, if allowed to remain, will cause a blister to form beneath, which is broken by friction, creating a painfully exposed area of true skin. In this event, the edges of thickened cuticle are cut away with the scissors, and an antiseptic dusting powder, such as aristol, sifted upon the wound to heal it.

After the removal of a soft corn, a Felt Disc or Washer is to be applied over it to prevent further friction or pressure. An old shoe should be worn several days until the parts have returned to a normal state.

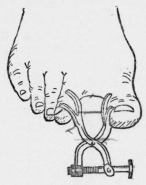

Fig. 41
TOE EXPANDER

If the feet perspire very freely, a condition often accompanying the presence of soft corns, they should be treated as later described. (See PERSPIRING FEET on page 58.)

VASCULAR CORNS.—This form of corn is not commonly encountered. Such corns are found mostly upon the sole of the foot, either under the heel or the ball of large toe. They resemble a wart, somewhat, and are composed of a number of small blood vessels from which they get their name.

These corns are of a spongy nature, lying deep in the skin and very little above it.

There may be a number of these vessels visible in the form of little red spots.

The skin about the corn is usually inflamed and tender.

The treatment for such corns is as follows: Prepare

the foot by bathing as for the removal of other corns, then carefully cut away with the corn knife or a corn file the upper surface, taking care not to incise or cut the veins. If the veins lie too near the surface to do this, or if a vein is cut in the paring treatment, touch the bleeding point with the dry tip of a lunar caustic pencil, or with a little nitric acid, applied with a wooden tooth pick. If the acid is used, be careful not to get it on the surrounding skin.

This at once causes the vessel to stop oozing, but nothing must be attempted further until healing has been established.

If there are a number of such red points showing, it is best to treat with nitric acid, applied to each spot with a toothpick. This is to be repeated every other day. In the meantime, place a chamois or a felt disc about the corn, in the manner previously described, to relieve pressure. Loose shoes are also advised.

After a number of such treatments, the corn will be found to grow smaller, or to shrivel up, finally disappearing altogether. The inflammation of the skin usually subsides in one or two days, if pressure on the foot is relieved as directed.

The discs of chamois or felt should be worn over the site of the corn for several weeks, even if there is no sign of the corn, to prevent its return and to give the skin an opportunity to become normally thick again.

CALLOSITIES OR CALLOUS SKIN.—This is a common condition of the feet, and is due to the friction of ill-fitting shoes. It usually appears in spots about the sole of the foot, at the heel, or the ball, or at both places. There may be one or more of such areas of thickened, horny skin closely grouped.

To restore these painful surfaces to a proper state
the foot is bathed as described heretofore. When dried,
the foot is taken between the fingers and the thumb of
the left hand, and the skin is pared or shaved off carefully with the scalpel, held in the right hand, as shown
in Fig. 42.

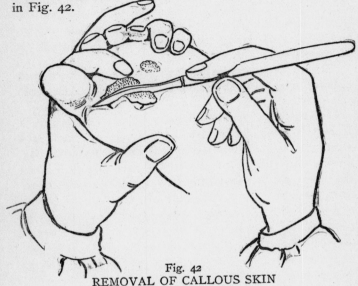

Fig. 42
REMOVAL OF CALLOUS SKIN

Do not cut carelessly, or too deep. Avoid wounding
the skin. Pare the callous down until the surface looks
pink and is thin to the touch.

It is well now to apply some antiseptic lotion, such as
listerine, or witch hazel. Allow this to remain on and
dry in, as it were. Dust on some stearate of zinc and
cover over the surface with a fairly thick layer of absorbent cotton. Over this lay a two-ply piece of borated
gauze and hold the whole in position with strips of rubber
adhesive plaster.

Advise the patron to wear a loose shoe. Owing to the movement in walking, these dressings are likely to be displaced and need to be renewed every day.

After the skin has taken on a more normal appearance, apply borated white vaseline to the area with a thin layer of cotton over it, and with gauze held in place by plaster strips. This tends to help nature restore the skin and to keep it soft and pliable at the same time.

ONYXIS, OR INGROWTH OF THE TOE NAILS.—This extremely painful condition is due to the careless cutting of the toe nails and the wearing of shoes narrow at the toes, or of shoes that, while broad enough, may press down too closely on the toes. The outer or inner sides of the great toe nail are usually affected, although any toe may be.

The skin of the sides of the nail, having been pinched against the nail edge continuously for weeks or months, soon rises over the nail and becomes thickened and swollen. Eventually the nail cuts into the groove thus formed, causing the most excruciating pain upon walking or even when standing quietly.

Some persons have a tendency toward ingrown nails because of the natural curvature of the nails, which, not being trimmed properly, soon grow down into the cuticle. It is therefore necessary in all cases to look very carefully to the trimming of the nails. The dry scales of cuticle should be removed from under the edges of the nail. The nail should be cut square across at its free end, and if, owing to a natural curvature of the nail, the edge tends to turn down at the sides, they should be elevated as hereafter described, and kept in this position until the nail ceases to curve downward. In the meantime the centre of the nail from the cuticle to the outer edge should be filed down. This tends to raise the sides of the nail.

Another method is, to cut a V-shaped piece out of the free edge of the nail. In doing this, care should be taken not to injure the tender skin under the nail. The filing down of the nail is shown in the dotted lines and the V-shaped cut in dark outlines in Fig. 43.

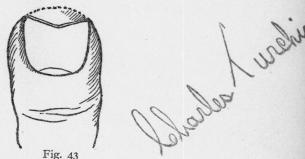

Fig. 43
FILING THE NAIL

If the nail sides have already curved downward, the dead scales of cuticle are removed carefully from under the edges with a pointed orangewood stick. This is followed with a packing of absorbent cotton, that should be allowed to remain there for twenty-four hours or two days, when it must be removed and replaced. This procedure should be continued until the nail has taken on a normal growth.

If inflammation or wounding of the skin has taken place, the treatment must vary accordingly. The foot should be bathed in hot water to which a teaspoonful of borax has been added. This softens the nail and skin and is antiseptic as well. The foot is now dried, and the parts about the ingrown nail are washed with a swab of cotton, dipped into listerine or alcohol, or into

a solution of peroxide of hydrogen and water, equal
parts.

The latter is especially useful, if pus has appeared at
the seat of irritation.

The peroxide will cause foam to appear at the site
of the wound. This is washed off with listerine, and

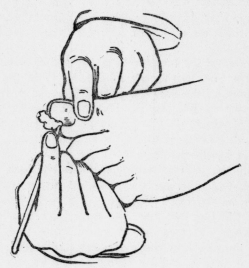

Fig. 44
INSERTING COTTON UNDER NAIL

the edge of the nail is pried up gently and out of the
inflamed groove. This will be found to be very painful,
and the entire lifting may not be accomplished at the
first sitting. If not, it should be repeated the next day—
and daily thereafter until the nail edge lies free above
the skin. In the meantime, a piece of absorbent cotton
is packed under the edge of the nail to keep it raised.
The method of introducing this is shown in Fig. 44.

A little zinc ointment should be applied to the inflamed skin and groove, to heal the parts. All pressure at the side of the toe should be avoided.

Another good method is to use a thin wedge of cork, which has been dipped into a weak carbolic acid solution before using. Two drops of carbolic acid to the ounce of water will answer very well. The advantage of the cork is that, as it becomes moist, it swells gradually and this raises the nail edge. This should be renewed every second day.

Either of the treatments is, of course, to be continued until a cure has been established. If in the meantime the edge of the nail appear rough or sharp, it should be trimmed of its jagged edges, which will give a great deal of relief. But much cutting is not advisable, since it tends to make the nail grow thick in some cases, and brittle in others.

The nail during treatment should be filed down thin along its centre, and the V-shaped cut be continued and made as shown in Fig. 43.

If the ingrown nail has caused too much skin disturbance, indicated by the parts being highly inflamed and swollen, and the nail edge has become so deeply buried that it will be found useless to pry it upward without causing damage to the toe, the patron should be advised to see a surgeon for a permanent operation in order that complete relief may be secured as quickly as possible.

BUNIONS.—If the foot has been subjected to the continuous pressure of a short or a too narrow shoe for a long time, it often happens that the skin over the second joint of the great toe at its outer side becomes inflamed. This may also happen on the outer side of the same joint of the small toe, or both great and small toes may be involved. This condition is, however, most commonly found in the large toe.

If this inflammation is not relieved, it leads, at first, to the formation of a callous, which, by the continued pressure, causes irritation of the *bursa,* or little sac that covers the joint cushion-like, to protect its delicate joint lining.

The inflammation under consideration at first leads only to a callous formation, disappearing in from three to four days when the cause is removed, but necessarily recurring at short intervals if the proper shoe is not placed upon the foot, and eventually leading to a thickening of the entire tissue about the joint, and then to an enlargement of the joint, and ultimately to a partial dislocation of the joint, the toe being thrown inward and forward, disfiguring the entire foot.

This condition must not be confounded with gouty or rheumatic disease. The history of the bunion is quite easily followed, and the gradual development of the enlargement, with spasmodic inflammation following the wearing of new or tight shoes, should convince the pedicurist of the correctness of his diagnosis.

The early relief and obliteration of a bunion is a simple matter, but once it has become chronic little can be done as a rule to give permanent relief except a surgical operation.

Given an early case of bunion during the stage of inflammation, all causes of pressure must be removed. Shoes of ample length and width across the ball of the foot should be advised at once. The foot should be bathed in hot water for fifteen to thirty minutes to reduce the inflammation, and a soothing lotion be applied over night to relieve the pain and swelling.

The following should be painted upon the part several times a day with a camel-hair brush:

R   *Tincture of Iodine* .... *2 dr.*
     Carbolic Acid .... *2 dr.*
     Glycerine .... *2 dr.*

Or, if the pain is very marked, the following may be employed with better result:

R   *Tincture of Belladonna* .... *2 dr.*
     Tincture of Iodine...................... *2 dr.*

This is painted about the joint at least three times a day.

After the bath, usually given at night, all callous skin and the small corns about the size of a split pea that are so commonly found about the enlarged joint should be trimmed away with the knife before the application of either of the above recipes is made.

If, by any chance, the skin is wounded, neither of these lotions must be used.

In such case, where the inflammation is moderate, a paste made as follows will be found to give relief:

R   *Zinc Oxide Powder* .... *2 dr.*
     White Vaseline .... *2 dr.*

Rub the vaseline and the zinc together well to make a smooth mixture. Apply to joint with two folds of gauze, over which place a layer of absorbent cotton, which must be held in place with strips of adhesive plaster.

Shoes should not be worn at any time during such treatment, or, if they must be, that part of the shoe over the toe joint should be cut out to relieve all pressure. A heavy stocking should then be used to cover the dressing just mentioned.

Hot or cold applications of witch-hazel at night often give excellent results in mild cases.

Once the inflammation, swelling and pain has subsided, do not let the patron wear a shoe without encircling the site of the bunion with a ring of felt, or chamois, to prevent further pressure on the part. See Fig. 45.

The faithful use of such a protective, and the wearing of proper shoes will usually effect a cure, if the case has been seen early enough.

If the case has become chronic or an abscess has devel-

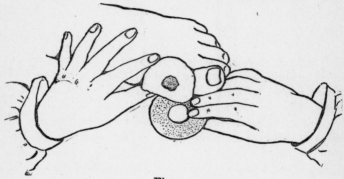

Fig. 45
APPLYING BUNION SHIELD

oped, a great deal of attention is required, and in most cases the services of a surgeon are necessary.

In case an abscess has formed, it is well to poultice the part with a flaxseed meal poultice, applied hot, at short intervals, until the skin becomes thinned out by the pressure of the pus, when it should be opened and the pus let out. The small lancet with which the incision is made should be sterilized both just before and after each operation by dipping into a little jar of sterilizing fluid.

The wound is washed with equal parts of peroxide of hydrogen and water, after which aristol powder is dusted on. Over this, lay two plies of gauze covered with absorbent cotton and a bandage to prevent infection or injury. This dressing is to be renewed each day.

Once the parts are healed, a protective bunion-shield or ring must be placed over the affected parts until recovery is confirmed beyond a possibility of relapse. Proper shoes, of course, are to be worn.

For dislocation of the toe, and enlargement of the joint, nothing but surgical intervention will be of any use. The patron must in this case be referred to a skilful physician or specialist.

FLATFOOT.—When the arch of the foot becomes weakened or broken down, the sole of the foot, instead of being arched between the ball and heel of the foot, becomes flat or sprawled.

This condition is becoming more and more marked in modern times, due principally to the wearing of improperly made shoes.

High heels are a cause to a great extent, as well as improperly balanced shoes with little or no support under the arch.

It is also caused by continuous standing, or by excessive walking or by adiposity. Even moderately stout persons are very liable to become victims of this affliction. Long-continued confinement to the bed, as during a protracted illness, or general weakness, are also causes. In such cases, the muscles of the leg having become weakened, the whole weight of the body falls upon the body structure of the foot, and causes it to give way.

Children who are taught to walk too early in life often become flatfooted.

The loss of the arch of the foot may occur at any time in life, and as often in men as women. It may be found more often with the former, however, in certain localities, where a man is subjected to long periods of work in a standing position, and eats improper or poorly cooked food. Low vitality and poor environment may be stated as very common causes.

The early symptoms of flatfoot are rather uncertain. There is no sign of inflammation about the feet. The patron complains of pains in the feet, a dull aching in the calves of the legs, and of becoming easily tired on standing or walking.

On examination the arch may seem to be as shown in Fig. 27, but as these symptoms continue to grow worse, and walking becomes a burden, the arch will be seen to fall lower and lower, until the entire sole of the foot falls flat upon the floor as shown in Fig. 28.

Once this condition has resulted, there is little possibility of restoring the arches to the normal position.

Cases must be recognized and treated early, in order to attain any marked relief, and, unfortunately, the patients will not often present themselves until too late.

Early in the disease, the feet should be bathed nightly in a hot bath to which a handful of sea-salt has been added. The bath should last about fifteen minutes. After thoroughly drying the skin, rub the feet with alcohol and have the patient go to bed so as to remove all strain from the feet.

Properly fitted shoes must now be provided. The heels should not be high, for, while very high heels at first seem to give relief, they only hasten the final ruination of the arch. Laced shoes, because they can be more simply applied to the feet, are best.

ARTIFICIAL ARCHES.—Arches of steel covered with leather have been much in vogue. They are bad. Arches of cork with a small steel spring have been tied to the feet and worn inside of the shoes, and are much better, but the cork becomes damp and swells and rots. If a glove of some kind that would resist dampness were put over them in making, the cork arches would be preferable for many feet. The arches now most in use and most advisable are of hard rubber with a small steel spring. These have a considerable elasticity, which the steel arch lacks, but they are liable to snap. These arches should be worn but an hour or two during the first and second week especially, because if they force the arch up abruptly they will cause great pain. They should be worn a few hours each day until the feet have become accustomed to them and the bones have begun to assum a position *near* that of the original.

In such cases, these arches should not be given up for years, inasmuch as the old trouble is apt to recur.

In severe cases a flannel bandage should be put on the feet after the bath at night; or Faradic electricity for ten minutes be applied to the feet before the bandages. These bandages are to be removed in the morning and proper shoes with arches worn. The sufferer should avoid standing for any length of time, and rest the feet as much as possible.

The treatment just suggested should be repeated every other day for several months to gain any benefit.

As a rule, all treatment in chronic cases gives only relief, since the arches once entirely broken down can rarely be replaced. The patron is therefore compelled to treat the feet with continuous care for the rest of life. If he or she can be taught by the chiropodist to realize early the importance of wearing sensible, well-fitting shoes and to adopt the use of proper arches therein, much good will result, because much ill will be escaped. Neglect of flatfoot eventually leads to intense physical pain and mental anguish that at times seems almost unbearable. Therefore, if you have cause to suspect from an examination of a patron's feet that flatfoot is likely to come, or if the stoutness of your patron indicates a liability to a sudden attack of it, advise earnestly against the dangers of neglect. The gratitude of an intelligent patron whom you have saved in time, or whose feet you have set right in the early stages of this common malady is often very great and constant.

CHILBLAINS.—Some persons are especially susceptible to frost bite or chilblains of the feet. Lowered vitality, snow water, severe cold and too quick heating of cold feet are the usual causes of chilblains.

At the first symptom, which is usually an itching of the foot, applications of olive oil or almost any handy grease should be put on without much rubbing. After the grease has been gently manipulated into the skin and between the toes, the surplus may be wiped off to avoid too much soiling the stockings. Care must be exercised to keep the feet dry, that is, thoroughly wiped or patted dry after bathing and wiped dry and the stockings frequently changed if the feet perspire.

Some persons appear to be particularly susceptible to chilblains, even a chill dampness causing the condition.

In some cases, the frost bite results in the loss of one or more toes.

When the case is seen early the feet should either be rubbed with snow until the circulation is re-established, or be placed into a cold bath which is warmed gradually. Any sudden application of heat is to be avoided. Even the room in which the patient is to be treated should be cool, so as not to increase the general circulation too readily.

To relieve any further discomfort, after such a bath or snow rub paint the chilblains with pure guaiacol. Repeat the external use of this several times during the day.

If the frost bites are not severe, they may be painted with equal parts of camphor and belladonna liniment, or with this:

R   Oil of Cajeput .... 2 dr.
     Strong Liquid Ammonia................. 2 dr.

Compound soap liniment enough to make 3 ounces.

If the skin over the parts has become cracked and sore, apply a soothing antiseptic ointment, such as the following:

R   Ichthyol .... 20 drops
     Zinc Oxide .... 1 dram
     White Vaseline .... 2 ounces

Mix into an ointment, apply on pieces of lint, and cover with absorbent cotton, or this, applied by binding on the part absorbent cotton or linen bandages soaked in it:

R   Glycerine .... 1 oz.
     Tincture Iodine .... 20 gr.
     Tincture Opium .... 20 gr.

To prevent further danger from frost bite, have the patient wear woollen socks or stockings. The use of an artificial perforated medicated insole is often helpful, as it also is in case of callosities,

Use a hot footbath, to which a handful of sea-salt has been added, each night, and follow after drying with an alcohol rub. Spirits of camphor are also soothing, or a mixture of half alcohol and half spirits of camphor may be used after the bath.

When there is intolerable itching or burning, this mixture applied on cotton or bandages to the parts often quickly soothes:

℞   *Burnt Alum* .... 5 *gr.*
      Iodide of Potassium..................... 2 *gr.*
      Laudanum .... 2 *gr.*
      Rose Pomade .... 5 *gr.*
      Lard (fresh)............................. 3 *gr.*

A so-called passive movement or treatment of the soles of the feet is to cross the foot over the opposite knee and with a ruler or short stick strike the sole of the foot a series of rapid light blows, about 30 or 40. The sole of the foot to be protected by a slipper. The benefit derived chiefly belongs to the capillaries and nerves of the part, the congestion of the capillaries, as in chilblains, is quickly scattered. The movement warms the feet and the cure of chilblains is often speedy and permanent.

Avoid placing the feet upon oven-hot air registers, or putting them near to the fire. Improve the health by proper exercise and food.

Perspiring Feet.—While perspiration of the feet is natural, excessive perspiration is a disease depending upon lowered nerve tone in the skin of the feet, or upon general poor health.

To overcome the condition improve the health first of all by proper living and food, healthful exercise, and daily care of the feet as heretofore prescribed.

For the sweating, the following powder will be found locally excellent:

℞   *Perborate of Soda* .... 1 *dr.*
      Salicylic Acid .... 20 *gr.*
      Boric Acid (powdered)................. 2 *oz.*

Mix the powders together well and shake about a teaspoonful into the shoes each morning.

Change the stockings each day, as well as the shoes, wearing each pair alternate days.

Another excellent powder is made of the following:

℞ Alum (powdered) .... ½ oz.
   Orris Root (powdered)............... 1 "
   Rice (powdered)..................... 2½ "

Mix well together and dust into the shoes as the above. The following, dusted on freely, will also be found excellent:

FOR PERSPIRING FEET

℞ Borax .... 10 grams
   Starch .... 10 "
   Salicylic Acid .... 3 "
   Powdered Alum .... 5 "
   Talcum Powder .... 50 "
   Naphthol 5

or this far simpler preparation often very quickly effective, can be applied with a camel-hair brush or soft sponge:

℞ Distilled Water .... ½ qt.
   Bichromate of Potassium.............. 1½ dr.
   Essence of Violet .... 1 dr.

If the patient suffers from excessive ill-smelling sweating of the feet, the following will be found highly satisfactory:

℞ Bismuth Subnitrate .... ½ oz.
   Permanganate of Potash.............. 6 dr.
   Rice Powder .... 1 oz.

Mix well and dust into the stockings and into the shoes, following the same general directions for the proper care of the feet as heretofore given.

HOT FEET AND CRACKS BETWEEN TOES.—If the cracks between the toes are caused by excessively hot feet, quick relief is obtained in most cases by a prompt application of zinc ointment over the cracked surfaces, or by powdering thickly with Fuller's earth.

If the feet are bathed nightly in tepid salt water or water into which a little borax has been sprinkled, there is little likelihood of sensitive swollen feet, or of hardened or calloused spots. Be careful when bathing the feet to dry between the toes thoroughly.

Rub any swollen portions of the feet with witch hazel or alcohol, and any hard, calloused places with olive oil or cold cream.

THE following books by **William A. Woodbury, Dermatologist,** now published, may be obtained from booksellers everywhere.

They are in the nature of Text-books and are written and illustrated with a view of providing, in a concise and authoritative manner, the methods for the care of the person that may be practiced by those who desire a working knowledge of Beauty Culture, either for self-improvement, or as a dignified means of money-making.

I. Hair Dressing and Tinting

A Text-book of the Fundamental Principles, Showing the Ready Adaptability of the Ever-changing Mode of Wearing the Hair.

For Professional and Private Use

Cloth Bound *Illustrated* *Price 50 cents*

II. The Care of the Hair and Scalp

How to Keep the Hair from Falling Out or Turning Grey.

A Text-book for Professional and Private Use

Cloth Bound *Illustrated* *Price 50 cents*

III. The Care of the Hand

A Practical Text-book on Manicuring and the Care of the Hand.

For Professional and Private Use

Cloth Bound *Illustrated* *Price 50 cents*

IV. The Care of the Face

How to Have Clear, Healthy Skin and How to Eradicate Blemishes of Face and Features.

A Text-book for Professional and Private Use

Cloth Bound *Illustrated* *Price 50 cents*

V. The Care of the Foot

A Practical Text-book on Chiropody and General Care of the Feet

For Professional and Private Use

Cloth Bound *Illustrated* *Price 50 cents*

VI. How to Get Thin and How to Acquire Plumpness

A Text-book for Professional and Private Use

Cloth Bound *Illustrated* *Price 50 cents*

G. W. DILLINGHAM COMPANY
PUBLISHERS NEW YORK